The Pritikin Diet for Beginners

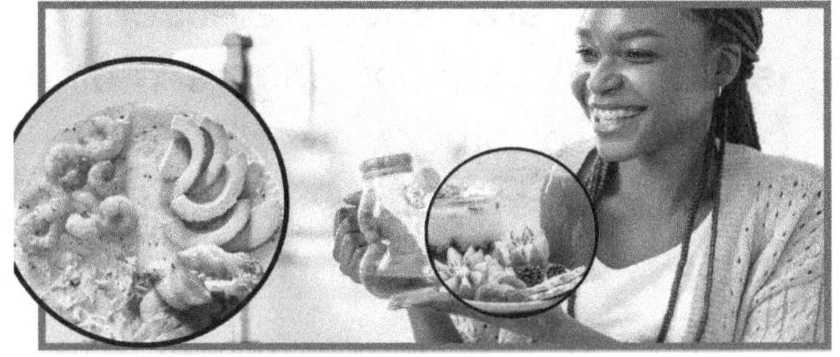

Elevate Your Fitness Journey with Comprehensive Menu Plans, Nutritious Recipes, and Proven Exercise Regimens for Weight Loss and Optimal Health!

Dr. Linda Wilson

Table of contents

Introduction

John D. was a middle-aged man who revered fry food, rosy meat, cheese, and butter.

He never cared about his prosperity until one day he went to the doctor for a planned checkup and got shocking news.

He had dangerously high cholesterol levels and was at risk of having a heart attack or stroke.

The doctor incited him to change his eating propensities and way of life.

Or else he will have to take pharmaceuticals for the rest of his life.

John D. was reluctant to give up his favorite supplements, but he too didn't need to depend on pharmaceuticals.

He has chosen to look for typical ways to lower cholesterol.

He looks online and finds a book called "The Pritikin Diet for Beginners," which claims to be an illustrated program to fight heart disease, diabetes, and weight gain.

Through a low-fat, high-fiber, plant-based slim down.

John D. was curious about the book and asked for a copy.

He read it carefully and learned that the Pritikin Diet calories are based on science and clinical examination, which has made a difference in thousands of individuals' prosperity and well-being.

The book also included equations, supper plans, and tips for remaining Diet.

John D. has chosen to allow it to be an endeavor.

He cleared out trash and food from his washroom and ice chest and ate normal items like vegetables, whole grains, beans, and nuts.

He also works out routinely, and each day he walks for at least 30 minutes.

To start with, he missed his old food and felt hungry and tired.

But he followed the book's rules, he took note that he had started losing weight, had more vitality, and was resting better.

He as well felt that his thrust was diminishing, and he got to be more confident.

Three months later, he returned to the doctor for a follow-up test. To his shock, he took note that his cholesterol levels had dropped through and through from 240 mg/dl to 160 mg/dl.

He also moved forward with his blood weight, blood sugar levels, and triglycerides.

The doctor was motivated and lauded him for his achievements.

He told him to keep up the awesome work, for which he didn't require any pharmaceuticals.

John D. was excited and communicated appreciation toward the doctor.

He guaranteed to continue with the Pritikin. Eat less and spread the word to his family and companions. He realized that he had found the key to a strong and cheerful life.

Welcome to the transformative journey of getting a handle on the Pritikin Tally calories! On this page, we delve into the pith of the Pritikin approach, understanding its roots and opening up the benefits that come with accepting this way of life.

Let's set out on a journey that goes beyond straightforward dietary choices, epitomizing thinking that progresses not in a reasonable weight incident but in common well-being.

What is the Pritikin diet of calories?

The Pritikin diet is more than a reasonable tally of calories; it's an all-inclusive way of life that pivots around making health-conscious choices. Built up by Nathan Pritikin, this approach emphasizes a tally of calories well off in whole, characteristic nourishments, coupled with standard workouts.

At its center, the Pritikin diet centers on finishing perfect prosperity by tending to the root causes of distinctive prosperity issues, such as down-and-out food and inert ways of life.

Understanding the beginnings and rationale behind the Pritikin diet is fundamental to getting a handle on its guidelines.

Nathan Pritikin, a nutritionist and life span examiner, made this approach in the late 1970s.

His reasoning was grounded in the thought that a check calorie deficit in fat and cholesterol, combined with working out, appeared expected and rearranged common, determined ailments.

The Pritikin diet is built on the foundation of overwhelmingly plant-based check calories, emphasizing aggregate grains, common items, vegetables, and slant proteins.

By diminishing the affirmations of drenched and trans fats, individuals taking after the Pritikin approach point to move forward heart prosperity, supervise weight, and overhaul by huge essentialness.

Benefits of the Pritikin Approach

The benefits of getting a handle on the Pritikin way of life are complex.

From weight incidents to cardiovascular prosperity, this chapter explores the positive influence of the Pritikin Tally calories on the body and judgment skills.

Consistent studies have consistently outlined the reasonability of the Pritikin approach for reducing cholesterol levels, bringing down blood weight, and progressing weight incidents.

Past the physiological benefits, the Pritikin Tally calories develop mental clarity and excited well-being.

The nutrient-dense nourishments recommended in this approach grant fundamental vitamins and minerals that support brain function, though typical exercise contributes to extending, diminishing, and advancing disposition.

Getting Started:

As you set out on your pilgrimage, understanding the key measures is crucial.

This range traces the significant rules that shape the bedrock of the Pritikin diet.

From choosing aggregate nourishments over taken care of choices to solidifying ordinary physical activity into your plan, these measures are arranged to be open for tenderfoots, though laying the establishment for persevering ways of life changes.

One of the central tenets of the Pritikin Diet is the emphasis on characteristic, common nourishments.

Whole grains, common items, and vegetables take center stage, providing essential supplements without the included sugars and disastrous fats found in various arranged nourishments.

Learning to consider food names gets to be an essential fitness skill, enabling you to make informed choices and avoid pitfalls in the cutting-edge food scene.

The Pritikin approach energizes cautious eating, savoring each snack, and paying thought to starvation and completion prompts. By developing a more significant affiliation with eating inclusion, individuals can form a more beneficial relationship with food, breaking free from the cycle of eager and neglectful eating.

In terms of physical development, Pritikin's thinking advocates for a balanced approach. This isn't brutal, tiring workouts; or maybe it emphasizes finding workouts you appreciate and can get back.

Whether it's brisk walking, swimming, or yoga, joining standard workout overhauls reaps, for the most part, the benefits of the Pritikin way of life.

As you acclimatize to the measures of this introductory chapter, you lay the foundation for a transformative journey toward prevalent prosperity and well-being.

The Pritikin diet isn't a reasonable or brief settlement; it's a temperate way of life that empowers you to take control of your prosperity.

So, let the journey begin, and may each step bring you closer to the energetic, eager life that Pritikin's thinking guarantees.

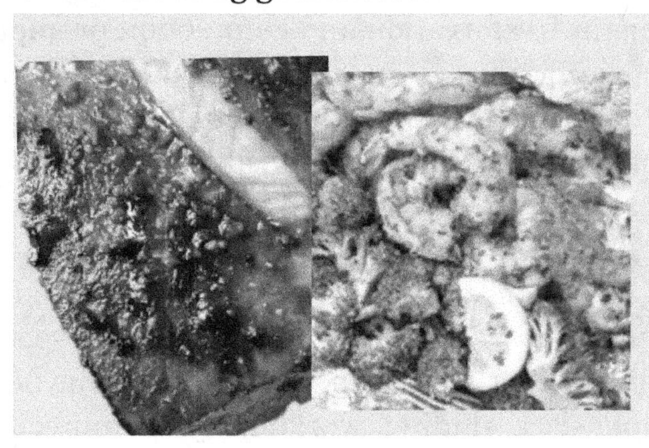

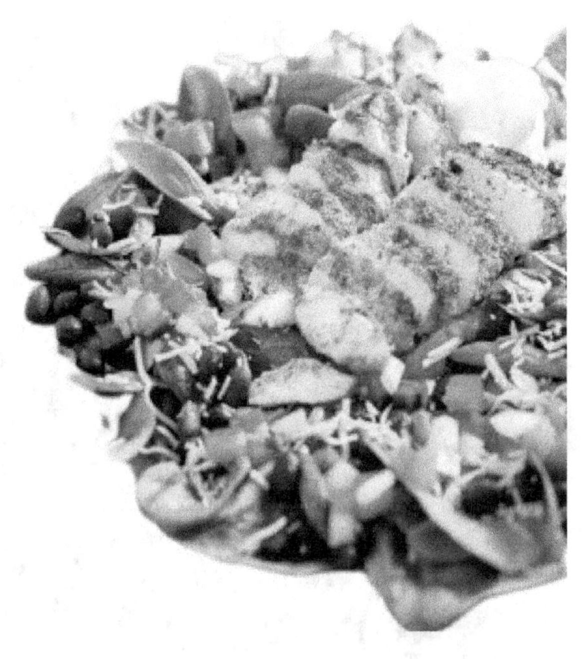

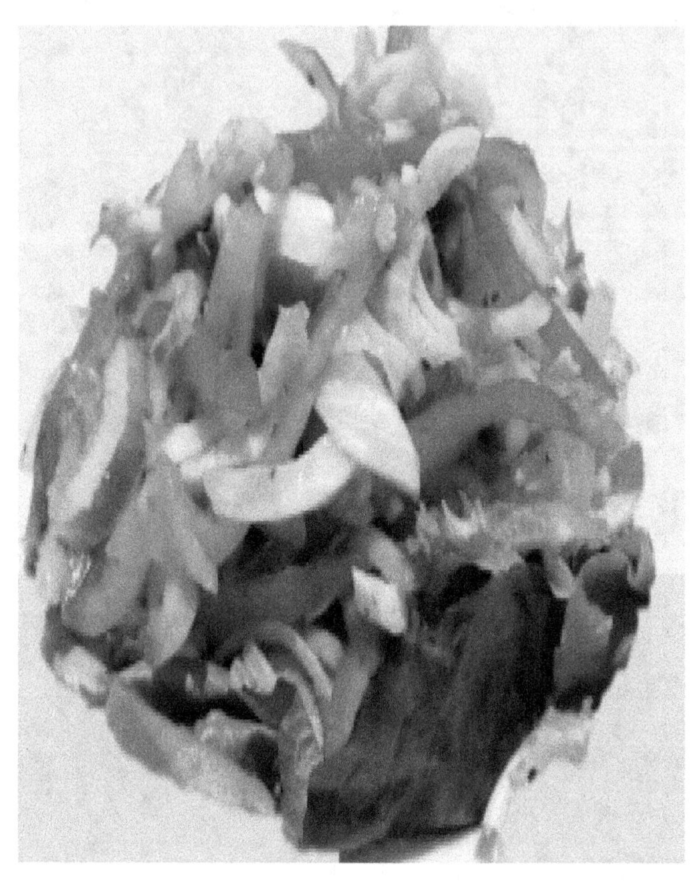

Chapter 1: Understanding Nutrition

This vital essay discusses the underlying nutritional theories that form the basis of the Pritikin Diet.

One must grasp the relevance of each nutrient and how it affects general health to make smart dietary decisions.

Let's review the principles of nutrient-dense diets, the relevance of lean proteins, the value of carbohydrates, and the acceptability of healthy fats.

Basics of Nutrient-Rich Foods

Meals that are substantial and rich in nutrients are the core of the Pritikin philosophy.

This covers the principle of nutritional density and why it matters to your health.

For every calorie, meals packed with nutrients provide a multitude of vitamins, minerals, and other vital components.

Fruits, vegetables, whole grains, and legumes take center stage as they are rich in health benefits and contain none of the empty calories found in diets that are processed. It becomes vital to grasp the relevance of micronutrients like vitamins and minerals.

These compounds are important for several biological activities, such as the immune system and bone health.

People who consume a diet high in a variety of colorful foods may make sure they acquire a wide range of nutrients essential for optimal health.

The Role of Carbohydrates in the Pritikin Diet

This essay attempts to address prevalent misunderstandings about carbohydrates in the nutrition business and explain their significance in the Pritikin Diet.

Contrary to widespread opinion, not all carbohydrates are created equal.

Common Pritikin method foods like fruits, vegetables, and whole grains provide complex carbs that give sustained energy without the fast blood sugar rises associated with processed carbohydrates.

By supporting readers in discerning between basic and complex carbohydrates, the chapter advises individuals to adjust their diets.

By consuming whole, unprocessed carbohydrates, people may regulate their blood sugar levels, feel full, and satisfy their long-term energy demands.

Embracing Healthy Fats

This dispels the misconception that all fats are harmful by highlighting healthy fats and their relevance in the Pritikin Diet.
While limiting overall fat consumption, boosting unsaturated fat sources—such as those found in avocados, nuts, seeds, and olive oil—is encouraged.
Knowing the difference
between unsaturated and saturated fats makes it vital to make smart nutritional decisions.

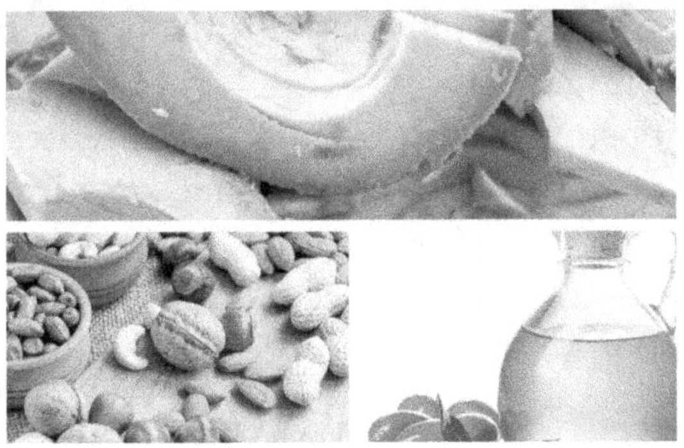

Consuming unsaturated fats has been linked to heart health advantages by reducing cholesterol and boosting cardiovascular health in general, according to a study.

When customers consume these healthy fats in moderation, they may still enjoy satisfying, substantial meals without jeopardizing their health goals.

This highlights the importance of lean proteins in the context of the Pritikin framework and the need for protein in a diet that is balanced.

Here, the emphasis is on acquiring your protein from plant-based sources like quinoa and tofu, as well as low-saturated-fat items like lentils, fish, and chicken.

This makes it easy for readers to comprehend how crucial protein is for sustaining muscle growth, general cellular health, and immune system function.

By choosing lean protein sources, consumers may achieve their nutritional requirements without worrying about the probable detrimental consequences of eating too much red and processed meat.

Readers who internalize the material from here will thoroughly comprehend the nutritional concepts of the Pritikin Diet.

This book covers everything from the relevance of nutrient-dense foods to the varied functions performed by carbohydrates, lipids, and proteins, offering readers the information they need to make educated and health-conscious dietary decisions. With this knowledge, employing the Pritikin approach to attain maximum health goes beyond following a diet and instead requires leading a robust and long-lasting lifestyle.

Chapter 2: Pritikin Meal Planning: Building Your Path to Health

On this page, we begin with a practical and vital part of the Pritikin Diet—meal planning.

This chapter is your guide to designing meals that match the principles of the Pritikin method, making it accessible and practical for anyone seeking a healthy lifestyle.

Let's walk through, covering planning balanced meals, mastering portion management, comprehending meal time, and presenting sample meal plans designed for beginners.

Building Balanced Meals

Creating balanced meals is the cornerstone of the Pritikin Diet, and here is your plan for success.

We study the notion of balancing macronutrients—carbohydrates, proteins, and fats—to ensure that each meal is nutritionally comprehensive and pleasurable.

This book includes practical ideas for including a range of colorful fruits and vegetables, complete grains, and lean meats into your meals.

By embracing diversity on your plate, you not only increase nutritious intake but also make your meals visually appealing and delectable.

This gives easy-to-follow suggestions for producing meals that fuel your body and pleasure your taste senses.

Building balanced meals is about producing a harmonic blend of nutrients that nourish your body and enhance general well-being.

In this book, we break down the components of a balanced meal:

carbs: Emphasizing whole grains, fruits, and vegetables, we underline the need for these complex carbs for sustained energy.

These foods give important fiber, vitamins, and minerals while avoiding the quick blood sugar rises associated with processed carbohydrates.

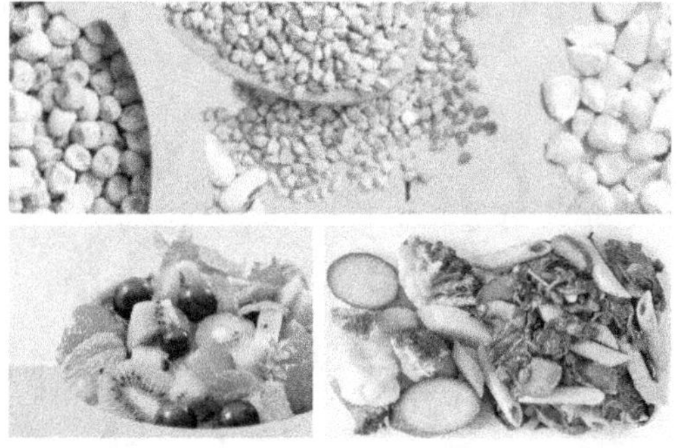

Proteins: Lean protein sources take center stage, with an emphasis on alternatives such as chicken, fish, lentils, and plant-based proteins. The chapter instructs readers on adopting these proteins to assist muscle maintenance, immunological function, and general cellular health.

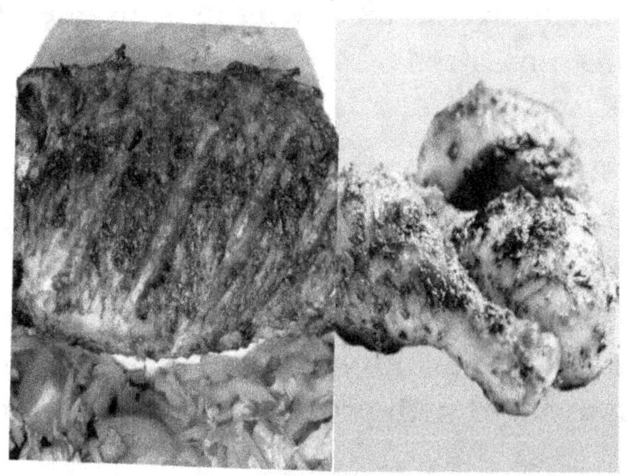

Fats: Healthy fats, such as those found in avocados, nuts, seeds, and olive oil, are incorporated to provide taste and fullness to meals.

Understanding the function of fats in a balanced diet dispels the misconception that all fats are deleterious, emphasizing the significance of moderation.

This presents realistic examples and easy-to-follow instructions, helping the audience to make meals that are not only nutritionally sound but also pleasurable.

Portion Control Strategies

Portion control is an important factor in the road toward a healthier lifestyle, and the article gives practical techniques to acquire this ability.

It highlights the need for mindful eating and understanding portion proportions to minimize overconsumption.

You will receive concrete ideas on utilizing smaller dishes, heed to hunger cues, and appreciating each bite.

By learning to understand the difference between portion sizes that satisfy hunger and those that lead to excess, individuals may take control of their eating habits and support their weight management objectives.

Portion management is typically a stumbling block in healthy eating, and this tackles the difficulty with effective strategies:

Mindful Eating: Encouraging readers to eat with awareness, relish each meal, and pay attention to hunger and fullness indicators.
By slowing down and being present at meals, individuals may build a healthy connection with food.

Smaller Plates: Utilizing smaller plates as a visual indicator for proper portion amounts.
This simple yet efficient method helps avoid overeating by naturally lowering the amount of food on the plate.

Smart Snacking: Offering tips on choosing nutrient-dense snacks and being cautious of portion choices between meals.
Healthy snacking is implemented as part of the overall plan to provide sustained energy throughout the day.

Meal Timing and Frequency

We go into the relevance of meal time and frequency, refuting popular misunderstandings and giving practical insights.

The Pritikin technique advocates a balanced distribution of meals throughout the day, maximizing energy levels and promoting metabolism.

You will understand the need for regular meal intervals and the possible benefits of avoiding lengthy periods without sustenance.

By having a consistent meal schedule, individuals can regulate blood sugar levels, limit the chance of unhealthy eating, and maintain sustained energy throughout the day.

This topic addresses the timing and frequency of meals, highlighting the following critical points:

Balanced Meal Distribution:

Advocating for a balanced distribution of meals throughout the day to avoid lengthy periods without food.
This technique maintains stable blood sugar levels and helps avoid unhealthy snacking or overeating during following meals.

Importance of meal: Highlighting the relevance of starting the day with a good meal to boost metabolism and supply critical energy for the day ahead.

Regular eating plan: Encouraging the audience to create a regular eating plan.
This regularity assists in managing appetite and improving digestion, leading to overall metabolic health.

Sample Meal Plans for Beginners

Putting theory into practice, this offers actual and realistic sample meal plans made exclusively for novices.

It includes a week's worth of meals, including different and accessible components that line with the Pritikin principles.

These example meal plans are not simply recipes but practical instructions, illustrating how to integrate Pritikin-approved meals into daily living.

From breakfast to supper, individuals may acquire inspiration and confidence in making meals that are both health-conscious and tasty.

This goes beyond theory, presenting real examples of what a week of Pritikin meals may look like for beginners:

Breakfast Ideas: Providing numerous and fulfilling breakfast alternatives, from whole-grain cereals with fruits to substantial omelets with veggies. These examples highlight the variety and versatility of Pritikin architecture.

Lunch Options: Featuring nutrient-packed meals, such as vivid salads with lean meats, whole-grain wraps, and comforting soups.
These meals are meant to keep you energetic throughout the day.

Meal Dishes: Offering delectable and health-conscious meal dishes, including lean meats, colorful veggies, and whole grains.
These examples illustrate that Pritikin meals may be both enjoyable and supportive of your health objectives.

Snacks and Desserts: Suggest sensible snack choices like almonds, yogurt, or fresh fruit, and explore dessert alternatives that accord with the Pritikin principles.
This emphasizes the concept that the Pritikin Diet is not about restriction but about making educated and pleasant meal choices.
As you absorb the lessons from this Topic, individuals not only comprehend the academic parts of the Pritikin Diet but also learn practical methods for applying this lifestyle to their everyday routine.
Meal planning becomes an easy and pleasurable chore, encouraging individuals to take ownership of their nutrition and begin on a path toward sustainable health and energy.

With balanced meals, regulated quantities, and smart meal scheduling, the path to wellness unfolds, one delicious and nutritious bite at a time.

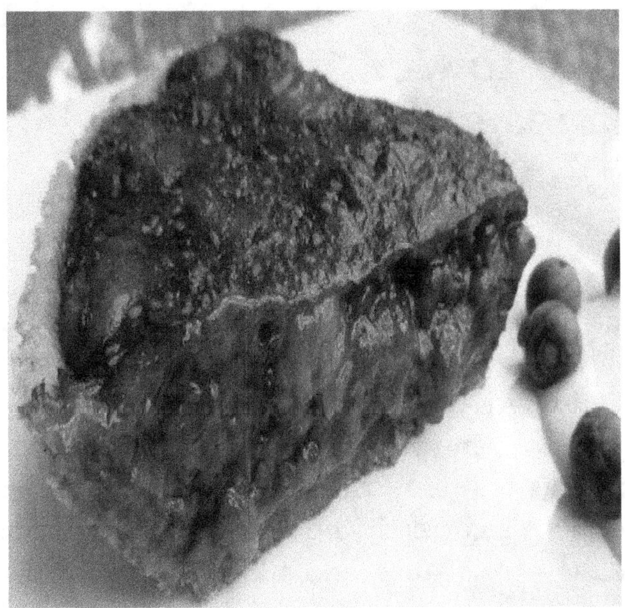

Chapter 3: Grocery Shopping Guide:

How to Get Around the Aisles for Pritikin Efficiently

Now, we apply the Pritikin methodology to real grocery stores in the real world.

This chapter is your comprehensive shopping guide to make sure the items in your basket are high in nutrients and suitable for Pritikin.

Let's look at this and learn how to identify products that are Pritikin-friendly, how to read food labels correctly, how to purchase sensibly, and how to organize a Pritikin pantry.

Identifying Pritikin-Friendly Foods

This can help you identify foods that follow the Pritikin Diet by acting as a guide for you while you peruse the aisles:

Produce Section: Highlighting the importance of consuming a wide variety of colorful fruits and vegetables.

This section provides practical tips on how to incorporate a variety of plant-based meals into your diet, pick fresh vegetables, and modify meal plans based on the season.

Whole Grains: Directing you to the parts of the nutritious grain group that include oats, brown rice, and quinoa.
Making decisions that support long-term energy and excellent health is made possible by understanding the distinctions between whole and processed grains.

Lean Proteins: When browsing the protein section, keep an eye out for lean alternatives like fish, fowl, lentils, and tofu.
Good advice on choosing high-quality proteins that align with the Pritikin worldview is readily available.

Healthy Fats: Look for products that are high in almonds, avocados, seeds, pecans, and olive oil in the aisles.
After this session, you'll feel ready and secure to include these fats in your meals for taste and satisfaction.

Study Food Labels Effectively

You must read food labels if you want Pritikin to work.

This book simplifies the process into simple steps:

Serving sizes: Explains how to assess serving sizes and adjust them to suit your individual needs.

This knowledge discourages unintentional overindulgence and encourages smart portion control.

Nutrient Content: To assist you in making selections, use the nutrition information panel to examine the primary nutrients.

This means recognizing the importance of fiber, staying away from added sugars, and cutting back on salt.

Ingredient List: Stressing the need to look for additives and preservatives that aren't on the list.

This enables you to choose meals that are as realistically close to their original state as possible.

Smart Shopping Tips

A Pritikin-friendly grocery shopping trip demands careful planning and selection of ingredients:

Meal Planning Before Shopping: Before going to the store, this technique advises viewers to create a shopping list that has all the products they'll need for healthful, well-balanced meals.

"Shopping the periphery" means telling customers to focus on the region surrounding the perimeter of the store, which is typically where lean meats, fresh veggies, and dairy goods are located.

This strategy cuts down on the amount of time spent eating processed and unhealthy food in the inner aisles.

Encouraging sticking to the shopping list and resisting the need to make impulsive purchases as a means of preventing impulsive expenditure.

This entails steering clear of visually appealing but nutritionally deficient items that are expertly arranged at eye level.

Putting together a Pritikin Pantry

The following assists you in stocking your Pritikin kitchen's pantry, which is its focal point:

Legumes with Whole Grains: Eating a variety of legumes, such as lentils and chickpeas, together with whole grains, such as quinoa, brown rice, and oats, is advised.

These are the main ingredients in meals that Pritikin approves.

Starting with heart-healthy oils is a great idea. Olive oil, for instance, is great for cooking and salad dressings.

This session examines how well Pritikin's emphasis on heart-healthy fats is supported by the items in your pantry.

Frozen or canned produce is considered a fair alternative to fresh produce.

This preserves the nutritional value while giving you more freedom to arrange your meals.

By the time you complete reading this chapter, you will know enough to support the Pritikin Diet by changing the way you buy at your local food store and by the way you behave.

This book equips viewers with practical knowledge on how to make informed, health-conscious shopping selections by teaching them how to select fresh fruit, read food labels, and plan meals.

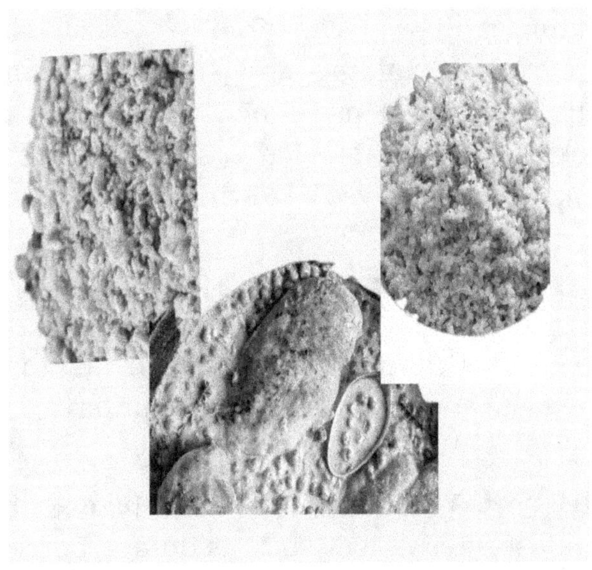

Chapter 4: Success Recipes for Pritikin Diet:

Tantalizing Treats on the Pritikin Plate

We explore the gastronomic facets of the Pritikin Diet on this page, offering a delectable selection of recipes that are sure to please.

This is a real treasure trove of scrumptious, high-nutrient dishes that show how tasty and fulfilling eating well can be.

Let's explore, talking about satiating dinner meals, nutrient-dense lunch alternatives, and snacks and sweets. Let's start with some breakfast alternatives à la Pritikin.

Delicious Breakfast Ideas

Here's some motivation in the morning to add some taste and nourishment to your day:

Whole Grain Delight: supplying filling breakfast alternatives such as quinoa porridge, nut butter, and toast with whole grains.

These options give you the nutrition and sustained energy you need to start your day with.

colorful and nutritious fruit meals that highlight the seasonal fruits' beauty.

These selections help you meet your daily need for vitamins and antioxidants while simultaneously satisfying your sweet tooth.

Serving inventive, high-protein egg dishes like poached eggs over whole-grain bread and vegetarian omelets is known as Egg-cellent Varieties.

Eggs are recognized by Pritikin as a versatile source of protein. These breakfast selections demonstrate this.

Mixed berries (strawberries, blueberries, and raspberries) and cooked quinoa

ingredients

Berry and Nut Quinoa Bowl.
- Diced almonds and walnuts
Greek-flavored yogurt
- Apply honey generously

Instructions

together with a big dish of mixed berries with cooked quinoa.

Top with Greek yogurt and chopped almonds.

-To make the bowl sweeter, add some honey.

Ingredients

Avocado and Vegetable Muffins: - Eggs

chopped cherry tomatoes, diced bell peppers, and spinach

Add salt and pepper to taste.

Instructions:

- Whisk together eggs in a bowl and season with pepper and salt.
- Stir in the diced vegetables.
- Muffin cups should be filled, and then baked until the mixture is done and the eggs are set.

Lunch Menu Selections Packed with Nutrients

Eating nutrient-dense meals that give you energy all day long makes lunchtime a joyful event:

A plethora of colorful salads made with succulent meats, succulent veggies, and delectable sauces are available to sample.

These salads are anything but ordinary; they combine a variety of flavors and textures to provide a filling and healthy noon meal.

Whole Grain Wraps: Presenting the taste and practicality of whole grain wraps stuffed with fresh vegetables, lean meats, and healthy spreads.

These travel-friendly selections offer a healthy balance of nutrients in each mouthful, making them ideal for people who are often on the go.

Hearty and calming soups prepared with veggies, lentils, and lean meats are available at Soup Sensations.

These soups are an excellent way to raise the comfort factor in your Pritikin lunch menu without sacrificing nutrients.

Mediterranean Chickpea Salad:

Ingredients

- Drained and rinsed chickpeas; - Diced cucumber; - Sliced Kalamata olives; - Crumbled Feta cheese; - Finely chopped red onion; - Lemon dressing with olive oil

Instructions:
- Combine the chickpeas, red onion, cucumber, tomatoes, olives, and feta in a bowl.
- Drizzle with the lemon dressing and olive oil, then toss to combine.

Grilled chicken wrap with quinoa:

Ingredients:
- A grilled chicken breast, sliced
- Mixed greens - Cooked quinoa - Whole grain wrap - Hummus - Sliced cherry tomatoes

Instructions:
- Spread hummus over the whole-grain wrap. Layer quinoa, cherry tomatoes, grilled chicken slices, and mixed greens.
- After wrapping, enjoy!

Satisfying Dinner Recipes

When you eat meals that both satiate your appetite and meet your nutritional demands, dinner becomes a gourmet experience:

Grilled Goodness: Have fun exploring the world of grilled chicken and fish paired with colorful veggie sides. These recipes show how using a grill to prepare food can be advantageous and tasty.

Plant-Powered Plates: Introducing plant-based supper alternatives that highlight entire grains, legumes, and veggies for their positive nutritional value.

These recipes highlight the variety of plant-based dishes and demonstrate how filling and substantial vegetarian dinners can be.

Discover how to stir-fry a variety of vibrant veggies and lean meats in Stir-Fry Wonders.

These dishes provide a tasty and easy way to add several kinds of nutrients to your evening meals.

Lemon juice and salmon filets

ingredients:
lemon-dill sauce fish.
- Finely chopped garlic Dill, freshly chopped; olive oil
Add salt and pepper to taste.

Instructions:
- Combine lemon juice, garlic, dill, olive oil, salt, and pepper to prepare a marinade.
- Let the salmon filets marinate for at least 30 minutes.
-The fish should be nicely done after baking or grilling.
Stir-fried veggies with tofu in them:

Ingredients
Cubed tofu, broccoli florets, sliced bell peppers, julienned carrots, snow peas, and low-sodium soy sauce ginger and garlic, minced

Instructions:
- Stir-fry the tofu for a golden brown color.
- Stir-fry the vegetables, garlic, and ginger until they are soft and crunchy.
- Drizzle with reduced-sodium soy sauce.

Desserts & Snacks the Pritikin Way

This satisfies your want for sweets and snacks without sacrificing your health objectives:
Nut-based foods, such as walnuts or almonds, are a satiating and nutrient-dense snack option.

You can get the protein and good fats from these selections to keep yourself full in between meals.

Fruit Infusions: Ingenious methods to serve fruits as snacks or sweets, either fresh or cooked in strange ways.
These choices highlight the fruit's inherent sweetness without using additional sugar.

Healthy Treats: providing Pritikin-approved desserts so you may indulge in sweets without compromising your efforts to be healthy.
Fruit sorbets and yogurt parfaits are just two examples of delectable treats that don't have to be unpleasant or guilt-inducing.

The Greek Yogurt Stand:

- Ingredients:
Greek yogurt
A range of fruits - Cereal - Drizzle with honey

Instructions:
- Add a mixture of berries, granola, and Greek yogurt to a glass.
- Proceed with the layers.
- Drizzle with honey before serving.

Banana nut oatmeal cookies:

Ingredients:
- Chopped nuts (walnuts or almonds) - Rolled oats - Mashed ripe bananas
- Cinnamon and vanilla extract

Instructions:
-Mash bananas, almonds, oats, cinnamon, and vanilla essence.
-Transfer the spoonfuls to a baking sheet and bake until golden brown.

By the time this book ends, you will have a newfound appreciation for the culinary options available within the Pritikin framework in addition to a variety of tasty dishes.
The goal of this session is to debunk the myth that eating healthily has to be monotonous or restricted by demonstrating how Pritikin meals can be a celebration of flavors and textures while encouraging the best possible health.

You may reap the benefits of culinary triumph on the Pritikin plate with the aid of this book, whether you're savoring a filling supper, a vibrant breakfast, a nutrient-dense lunch, or a guilt-free snack or dessert.

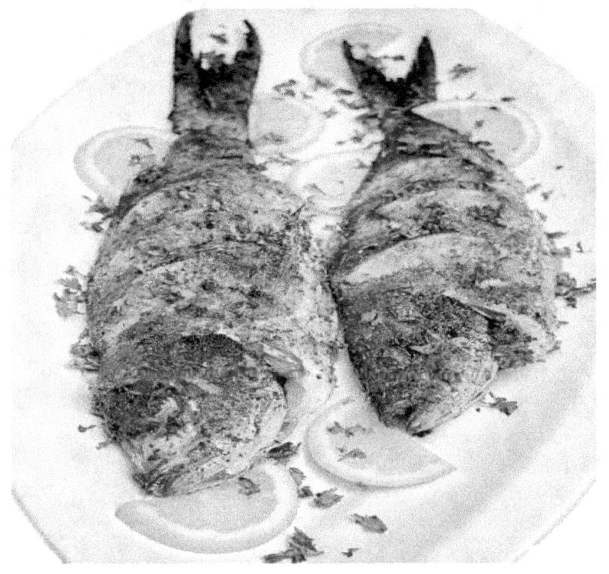

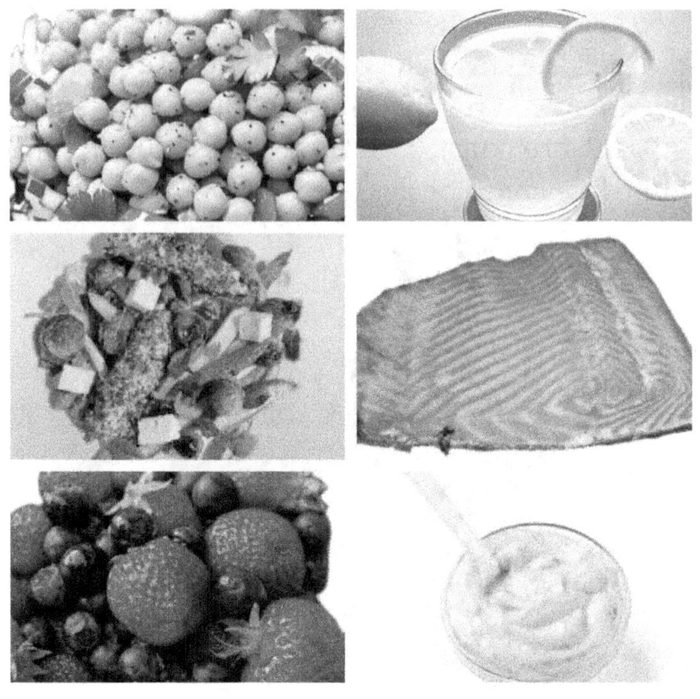

Chapter 5: Exercise and Fitness

Revival of Pritikin Way of Life

Moving from the kitchen to the living room or gym, we examine the value of fitness and exercise in the Pritikin way of life.

This chapter contains detailed information on how to include exercise into your daily routine to improve your general health and assist with weight management.

Let's get right to it and talk about how to get exercise into your daily routine, workout plans that are suggested by Pritikin, how to strike a balance between strength and cardio training, and the advantages of exercise for managing weight.

Including Exercise in Your Daily Routine:

No matter how busy or fit you are, here's how to squeeze exercise into your daily routine.

Daily Movement: The goal of raising the barrier for physical activity is to inspire viewers to engage in routine, daily activities that contribute to
This involves working exercise into routines like going for short walks, riding a bike, or using the stairs.

Setting Realistic Goals: emphasizing the need to establish realistic and reachable goals for exercise.
Whether your goal is to accomplish a daily step count or to gradually increase the intensity of your activities, setting reasonable targets may help you develop a long-lasting fitness habit.

Setting Realistic Goals: Stressing the importance of choosing fun hobbies for yourself.
You will probably go on with whatever activity you like, whether it is athletics, dancing, hiking, or something else.

Things that Pritikin sanctioned

The following exercises have been approved by Pritikin to promote flexibility and inclusivity:
Walk quickly to obtain the maximum benefit from this crucial and efficient cardiovascular exercise.
For individuals of all fitness levels, brisk walking, whether done outside or on a treadmill, improves heart health and burns calories.

Benefits of Swimming: as a full-body exercise.
Since swimming is easy on the joints and strengthens the heart, it's a fantastic substitute for those with joint problems.

Stretching Exercises and Yoga:
These have been recommended as great ways to improve balance, flexibility, and calmness.
To improve overall health and suit different levels of fitness, these workouts may be modified.

Strength and Cardio Training

A well-rounded fitness regimen must strike a balance between strength and cardio exercises.
Cardiovascular Exercises: Discusses the benefits of heart-rate-raising exercises including cycling, running, and aerobic training.
more endurance, better cardiovascular health, and more calorie burning are just a few benefits of cardiovascular exercise.

Strength Training: Emphasizes the advantages of using weights, resistance bands, or body weight as a training technique.
Strength exercise increases metabolism, promotes the growth of new muscle, and improves overall functional fitness.

Funding a Balance: Highlighting the advantages of strength and aerobic training for overall health.

A well-designed program ensures that participants maintain and increase their muscle mass in addition to burning calories

Exercise's Function in Weight Management

It's critical to comprehend how exercise aids in weight management:

Caloric Expenditure: Exercise is the major way to create a calorie deficit, which helps with weight loss or maintenance.

Combining a Pritikin Diet with consistent exercise increases the effectiveness of living a healthy lifestyle overall.

Metabolism Boost: Describe how regular exercise increases metabolism and makes it possible to burn calories effectively even while at rest.

This increased metabolism aids in maintaining a healthy weight and overall vigor.

Long-term Sustainability: Stressing the long-term benefits of consistent exercise and how it promotes general health and weight control rather than short-term goals.

Readers will realize that exercise is an integral element of the Pritikin lifestyle, not something that exists independently of it.

People of all backgrounds and fitness levels may achieve fitness because it promotes realistic goals, enjoyable activities, and a balanced approach to strength and aerobic training.

This chapter offers helpful and entertaining guidance on using exercise as the cornerstone of your Pritikin journey and as a means of leading an active, healthy lifestyle.

Chapter 6: Getting Past Obstacles to Achieve Success on the Pritikin Journey

We are finding it challenging to get over the typical obstacles in our way of living the Pritikin way.

This chapter contains answers to frequently asked questions and common misconceptions as well as advice on controlling cravings, dealing with others in social situations, and maintaining motivation while following the Pritikin Diet.

Let's examine how we may make the journey appear doable and open to anyone.

Compromising with Others in the Public

Learn useful strategies to uphold your Pritikin commitment in social situations:

Communication Proficiency:

Develop your communication skills to confidently and effectively explain your culinary preferences.

Discover how to participate in discussions about food without coming out as forced or isolated.

Make Wise Meals Choices: Take into account advice on how to choose meals for social events attentively.
Seek methods to achieve your objectives while maintaining your social networks; some suggestions are to bring Pritikin-friendly food to potluck events or make wise choices at the buffet.

Organizing Forward: Recognize the value of anticipatory preparation.
You may make sure that Pritikin-approved meals are accessible when you need them, which will make following your diet plan easier, by making plans ahead of time and anticipating social activities.

Handling Cravings

Take on the problem of cravings by using sensible and doable strategies:

Recognizing Cravings: Learn about the science underlying cravings and how they are related to triggers that are both physical and emotional. You may effectively treat cravings by developing methods based on an awareness of the underlying reasons.

Conscientious Indulgences: Acquire the Mindfulness to Savor.
To sate your appetites without sacrificing your health objectives, look for substitutes that Pritikin has authorized.
You may enjoy snacks in a way that supports your general health by making educated decisions.

Accepting Variability: Realize how important it is to have diversity in your Pritikin recipes.
Including a variety of enjoyable things in your diet will help you feel less deprived and less inclined to reach for unhealthy options.

Sustaining Motivation During the Pritikin Diet.

To keep your excitement for the Pritikin way of life alive, employ these strategies for long-term success:

Establishing reasonable goals: Ensure that your trip is accompanied by reasonable, attainable goals.
Celebrate your small accomplishments to keep your spirits up on your trip to Pritikin.

Establishing a Support Network: Acknowledge the significance of a strong sense of community.
Having a support system of friends, family, or fellow Pritikin aficionados may offer sharing success stories, accountability, and motivation.

Monitoring Development: Utilize resources to monitor your advancement. Maintaining a food journal, writing down your fitness goals, or tracking changes in your energy levels are all ways to strengthen your resolve to live a Pritikin lifestyle.

Handling Common Issues and Imaginations

Address frequent worries and misunderstandings head-on by providing correct facts.

Harmonizing Elements: Recognize the significance of upholding a nutritious diet from Pritikin's point of view.

The variety and abundance of the meals permitted on the Pritikin Diet should allay worries about nutritional inadequacies.

The durability of the Pritikin Way of Life:

Examine if the Pritikin style of life is sustainable over the long run.

Dispel the myths surrounding starving by highlighting the variety of mouthwatering and filling dishes that adhere to the Pritikin Diet's guidelines.

Method individualization:

Acknowledge the distinctiveness of the Pritikin approach.

Stress that the Pritikin lifestyle's flexibility to accommodate a wide range of dietary requirements, tastes, and lifestyles makes it advantageous to a wide range of people.

Readers will feel prepared to face obstacles on their Pritikin path with a strong mentality and practical understanding after finishing this book. This chapter will assist people in adopting the Pritikin lifestyle in an efficient

and long-lasting manner by answering
questions, busting myths, overcoming cravings,
projecting confidence in social situations, and
staying motivated.

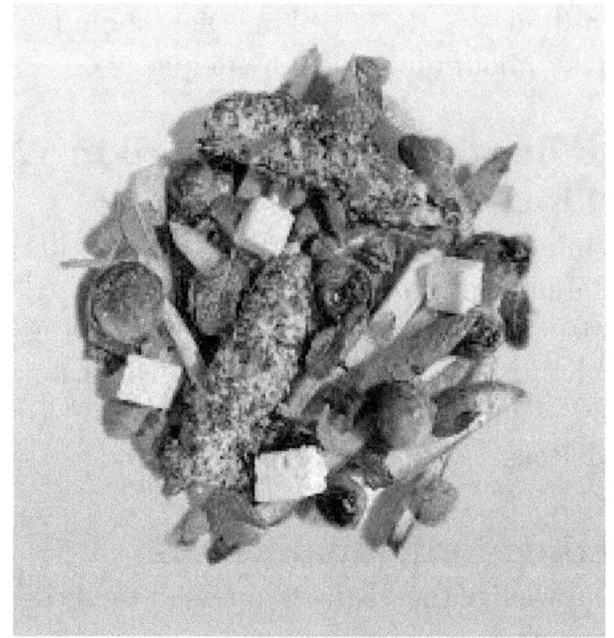

Chapter 7: Monitoring Development for Pritikin Achievement

We investigate the vital component of monitoring your Pritikin journey's development.

This component acts as your compass, offering helpful advice on how to set realistic objectives, track your weight and health indicators, recognize your accomplishments, and modify the Pritikin method for sustained success.

To make it simple and enticing for everyone to follow along, we will go over every aspect together.

Having Reasonable Objectives

Set measurable goals before you embark on your Pritikin journey:
Customized Objectives:

Recognize the significance of adjusting objectives to your particular situation.

Whether it's lowering cholesterol, losing weight, or having more energy, establishing attainable yet unique goals boosts motivation and achievement.

Both short- and long-term goals: Make a distinction between your short- and long-term objectives.
When aiming for more comprehensive, long-term results, setting more manageable goals helps one feel accomplished.

Including Lifestyle Modifications: Accept the notion that objectives go beyond the scale.
Make lifestyle modifications like consistent exercise, a mindful diet, and enhanced general well-being essential to your Pritikin goals.

Keeping an eye on health and weight metrics

Keep a careful watch on the following important health signs as you travel:

Frequent Weigh-Ins: Use frequent weigh-ins as a way to monitor your progress. Recognize that daily differences in weight are not abnormal and concentrate on general trends instead.

This gives you important information about how well your Pritikin lifestyle is working.

Metrics related to health: Expand to track more health parameters in addition to weight.
Check blood pressure, cholesterol, and other pertinent indicators regularly. These measurements provide a thorough picture of your health's development and the advantages of the Pritikin method.

Healthcare Professional Consultation: Understand the value of healthcare experts' consultation for a comprehensive evaluation.
Frequent check-ups guarantee that you will receive tailored advice and modifications to your Pritikin journey according to your specific health requirements.

Honoring Successes

Celebrate and acknowledge your small accomplishments along the way.
Acknowledge accomplishments that go beyond the scale.

Honor your improved mood, more energy, and general well-being as important indicators of your progress on the Pritikin path.

Organizing Milestone Celebrations: Plan milestone events to commemorate accomplishing particular objectives.
Rewarding yourself with wellness-focused items or a nutritious dinner at your favorite restaurant and recognizing your accomplishments strengthens your resolve to live a Pritikin lifestyle.

Sharing Success Stories: You might want to tell the Pritikin community, your family, or friends about your achievements. Sharing successes creates a positive atmosphere and motivates people to continue their health-related pursuits.

Modifying the Pritikin Method for Extended Achievement

Modify the Pritikin strategy to guarantee long-term success:
Flexible adjustments: Recognize that adaptability is essential for long-term success.

Adjust the Pritikin method to your preferences, changing circumstances, and changing health objectives, all the while being true to your dedication to total well-being.

Adapting and Learning: See your Pritikin experience as an ongoing educational process.
To achieve consistent, long-term success, iterate and improve your strategy in light of your experiences, learning what suits your body and lifestyle the best.

Constructing a Lasting Lifestyle: Put more emphasis on creating a lasting lifestyle than on making quick fixes.
Accept and incorporate the Pritikin principles into your everyday life as a basis for your ongoing health and well-being.

By the time this chapter ends, you will possess the resources to monitor their advancement with efficiency as well as the mentality to recognize accomplishments and make wise changes for sustained success.
This chapter serves as a testament to the Pritikin lifestyle's enduring qualities by highlighting the idea that measuring progress involves more than just arriving at a

destination—rather, it involves creating a lively and sustainable path toward long-term health and well-being.

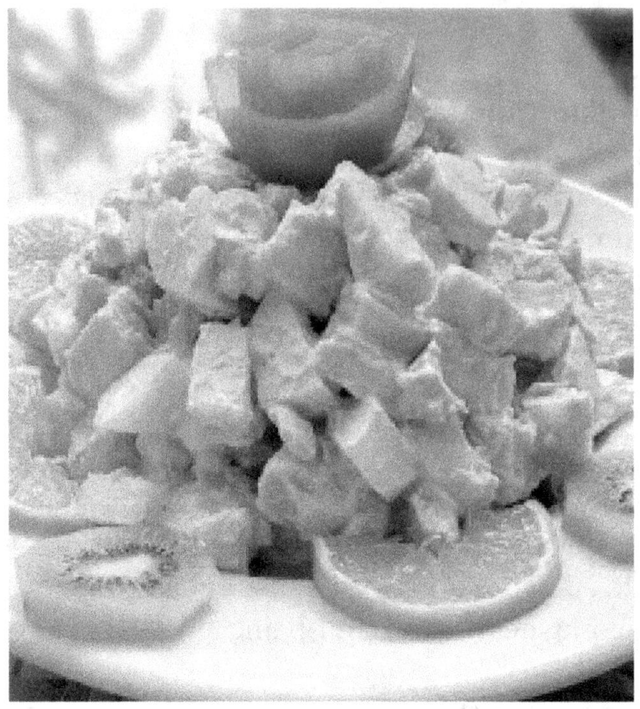

Chapter 8: Navigating FAQs and Troubleshooting on Your Pritikin Journey

You might have queries when you visit Pritikin. In this lecture, we explore typical questions and problem-solving approaches.

This comprehensive resource gives brief answers to commonly asked concerns, tips on overcoming hurdles and knowing when to visit a specialist, as well as data on medical conditions and dietary restrictions.

Let's check into this to make sure that everyone can grasp and find the information fascinating.

Responses to Commonly Asked Questions

Prepare thoughtful responses to the most typical inquiries regarding the Pritikin style of life:

Understanding Dietary Principles:

Read Grasp Dietary Principles to obtain a grasp of the core ideas underpinning the Pritikin Diet.

Describe how eating a diet rich in whole, nutrient-dense foods, avoiding salt, and sustaining the macronutrient balance are critical for achieving maximum health.

Navigating Specific Food Concerns: Address frequent inquiries surrounding certain foods including fruits, grains, and fats.
Encourage a diversity of food alternatives, healthier choices, and portion management by utilizing the Pritikin paradigm.

Balanced Nutrient Consumption: Explain how to maintain a Pritikin-compliant diet while making sure that the nutrients you take in are distributed effectively.
The relevance of moderation and diversity for a well-rounded nutritional profile cannot be emphasized.

Resolving Dead Ends

Overcome inactivity with practical techniques to continue moving forward:

Assessing Lifestyle issues: Consider lifestyle issues that may lead to plateaus.
Exercise, appropriate sleep, and stress management are vital.

They may examine and maximize various elements of their life by discussing these thoughts with others.

Reevaluating Food Selections: Help the viewer evaluate the food they have picked when they come to a halt.
Emphasize the benefits of maintaining a food journal, eating with awareness, and maybe adjusting meal selections and portion levels.

Including Difference: Emphasize that to go above dietary limitations, you must adjust your diet.
People should be encouraged to try different meals and dishes that Pritikin has permitted to nurture curiosity and development.

Looking for Professional Guidance

Recognize when you need to acquire specialist guidance by seeking expert help:

Getting Guidance from Medical Professionals: Stress the importance of visiting a medical practitioner.
Stress that doctors may supply personalized counsel depending on the demands and circumstances of each patient.

Registered Dietitian Support: You will promote the registered dietitian's role in making dietary advice by aiding them.
With the guidance of a nutritionist, patients may address concerns, construct tailored meal plans, and follow the Pritikin Diet for optimum outcomes.

Expert assistance from fitness specialists: When establishing tailored training routines, asking for help from fitness specialists is encouraged.
Exercise routines may be personalized by fitness specialists to each individual based on their aims and current fitness level, offering a comprehensive approach to well-being.

Taking Care of Nutritional Restrictions and Health Issues

Treat food limitations and medical difficulties with sensitivity and appropriate advice:

Adapting the Pritikin Principles: Explain how the Pritikin technique may be altered to meet individual dietary restrictions or health conditions. Emphasize how the Pritikin principles may be adjusted to each person's individual needs.

Collaborating with Medical Professionals: Stress the value of partnering with healthcare providers.
Promote frank communication about health problems and dietary limitations to ensure that the Pritikin technique corresponds with general well-being.

Examining Possible Modifications: Discuss alternate choices for people with unique dietary needs.
Make recommendations for alterations and substitutes that address particular health requirements while respecting the integrity of the Pritikin principles.

Readers will be better prepared to begin their Pritikin journey by resolving frequent inquiries, overcoming hurdles, getting expert help, and dealing with dietary limitations or health challenges after reading this section.
This component is vital for helping individuals grasp and move over problems, which makes it simpler for them to effectively adopt the Pritikin lifestyle.

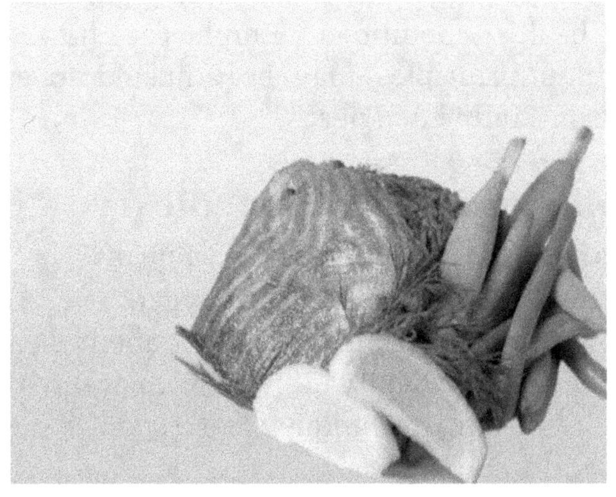

Chapter 9: Embracing Sustainability and Beyond in Your Pritikin Journey

We investigate the topic of sustainability within the Pritikin lifestyle and assist you beyond the early phases of adoption.

This session provides a path for making Pritikin a sustainable lifestyle, accepting incremental shifts, exploring advanced tactics, and motivating others via sharing your Pritikin story.

Let's look into it, to ensure clarity and accessibility for everyone.

Making Pritikin a Sustainable Lifestyle

Understand the keys to adopting Pritikin ideas easily into your regular life:

Creating routines: Emphasize the necessity of converting Pritikin methods into regular routines.

Discuss the importance of repetition and consistency in changing the concepts into a sustainable and natural part of your lifestyle.

Building Supportive surroundings:
Examine the role of your surroundings in sustaining the Pritikin lifestyle.
Foster a supportive home and work environment that supports healthy choices and reduces potential hurdles.

Enjoying the Journey: Shift the attention from short-term goals to the delight of the continuing journey.
Emphasize that Pritikin is not a fast fix but a lifelong commitment to health and well-being, with each day presenting a chance for positive choices.

Gradual Transitions and Adaptations

Navigate the process of incremental adjustments and modifications to achieve long-term success:

Introducing tiny improvements:
Advocate for the power of tiny, gradual improvements.
Encourage viewers to start with reasonable modifications, allowing the incorporation of Pritikin principles to be a gradual and sustainable process.

Adapting to Preferences: Acknowledge the flexibility of the Pritikin lifestyle. Emphasize that individuals may alter the method to fit their interests, ensuring that Pritikin stays a customized and pleasurable adventure.

Learning from obstacles: Discuss the inevitability of obstacles and failures. Encourage readers to regard these occasions as chances for learning and growth, emphasizing the resilience needed for a sustained Pritikin lifestyle.

Exploring Advanced Pritikin Strategies

Look at advanced tactics for individuals willing to take your Pritikin adventure to the next level:

Fine-tuning Nutrition Ratios: Explore the subtleties of nutritional ratios within the Pritikin framework.
Discuss how people may fine-tune their macronutrient consumption depending on their particular health objectives and reactions.

Optimizing Exercise regimen: Guide folks in optimizing their exercise regimen.

Discuss advanced fitness tactics, such as interval training or particular strength programs, for people wishing to better their physical well-being.

Incorporating Mind-Body activities: Introduce advanced mind-body activities, such as mindfulness meditation or advanced yoga methods.

These activities complement the Pritikin lifestyle, contributing to general mental and emotional well-being.

Inspiring Others: Sharing Your Pritikin Journey

Empower individuals to encourage and share their Pritikin experience with others:

Leading by Example: Emphasize the significance of leading by example.

Encourage individuals to embrace the Pritikin principles, displaying the good improvements in their own lives as an encouragement to friends, family, and communities.

Sharing Success Stories: Highlight the value of sharing success stories.
Whether through social media, community gatherings, or personal discussions, individuals may inspire others by sharing their Pritikin journey, achievements, and lessons gained.

Creating a Supportive Community: Explore the function of a supportive Pritikin community.
Encourage individuals to connect with like-minded individuals, building a feeling of community and sharing inspiration on their health and wellness journeys.

Upon reaching the last chapter, individuals will possess the tools to embrace the Pritikin lifestyle and access advanced tactics, enabling them to encourage others on transforming journeys.
This part functions as a guiding light, helping individuals toward a sustainable and rewarding Pritikin lifestyle, producing a ripple effect of good impact for both themselves and those in their orbit.

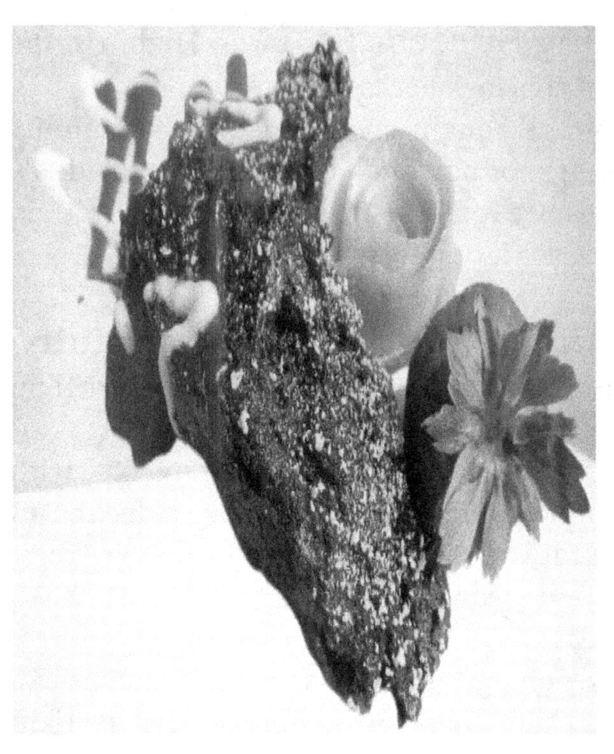

Conclusion:

Starting the Pritikin Diet and Traveling Through Life to Achieve Health.

As we approach the end of this introduction to the Pritikin Diet, it's crucial to recognize that what began out as a quest for better nutrition has expanded into a full way of life with the ultimate objective of enhancing your health.

The Pritikin approach blends exercise, mindfulness, community, and healthy nutrition into a sustainable and satisfying way of life. It is not just a diet.

We've gone over the Pritikin Diet's foundations, analyzed the significance of mindful living, and spoken about typical difficulties that may come up when you're attempting to improve your health via the chapters.

Every step toward a holistic approach to wellness—from defining realistic targets and evaluating your progress to breaking through plateaus and personalizing the Pritikin principles to your own needs—contributes.

The adaptability of the Pritikin lifestyle is what makes it so lovely.

The ideas are the same, promoting complete, nutrient-dense meals, physical exercise, and mindful practices, regardless of your degree of experience or desire to master advanced techniques.

This is a personalized journey that evolves as you do—it's not a one-size-fits-all plan.

As you begin out on this lifetime journey, bear in mind that your general well-being, enhanced energy, and better mood will serve as more accurate indications of success than the number on the scale.

The Pritikin way of living stresses forming resilient habits, recognizing the joys of everyday health, and developing sustainable lifestyle choices.

Think about the effect you can have on others in addition to your progress.

Your Pritikin journey, triumphs, and insights become a source of inspiration for everyone around you when you share them.

Positive decisions have a cascading effect that benefits the complete individual, building a community that is committed to wellbeing.

Adopting a Pritikin lifestyle requires more than just sticking to a diet; it includes adopting a way of thinking that puts your longevity, well-being, and the joy of living a complete life first.

Thus, embrace this as more than simply a plan; embrace it as a traveling buddy on your continuing trek to a happier, healthier life through the Pritikin Diet.

May well-being overflow from your path and that you urge others to go on this life-changing journey with you.

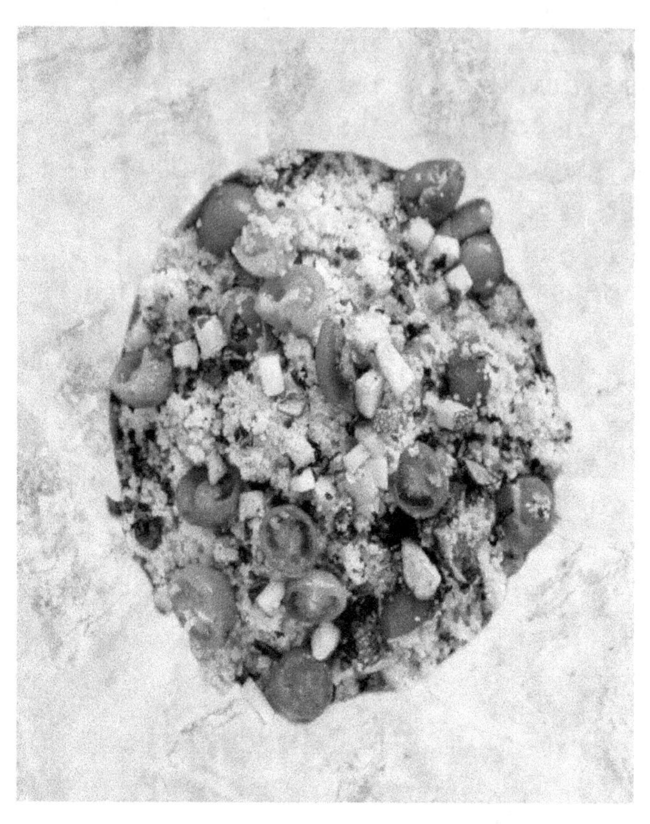

DIET PLANNER TIME TABLE

Day	Recipes	Remark
1		
2		
3		
4		

5		
6		
7		
8		
9		
10		

11		
12		
13		
14		
15		
16		

17

18

19

20

www.ingramcontent.com/pod-product-compliance
Lightning Source LLC
Chambersburg PA
CBHW061003260726
48661CB00005B/2017